Yoga:
The Essential
Guide

How to Master Weight Loss, Stress Reduction
and Find Inner Peace

M.E. Dahkid

ISBN: 1500171131
ISBN-13: 978-1500171131

DEDICATION

For those in search of a well-balanced exercise that activates the physical, mental, and spiritual realms within our bodies that promote healthy habits.

CONTENTS

	Introduction	i
1	Yoga Origin and Significance	1
2	How Yoga Promotes Weight Loss	5
3	Understanding Stress	13
4	Yoga Poses for Stress-Reduction	19
5	Yoga's Role in Finding Inner Peace	29
6	How Meditation is Beneficial for Yoga Practitioners	33
5	A Final Word	37

INTRODUCTION

I want to thank you for purchasing this book, "Yoga: The Essential Guide".

Over the last 20 years, the popularity of yoga has increased from nearly no interest to being one of the most popular exercise regimes around.

The objective of the yoga practice is to enable a man to reach a better understanding of one. Yoga helps one manifest and manifold the true expression of being Yoga is important because it is a well-balanced exercise that activates the physical, mental, and spiritual realms within our bodies that promote healthy habits.

Yoga is about balance, both mind and body, as well as increasing self-awareness, with by-products of better strength and flexibility. In the West, especially, yoga practice is typically focused on an asana practice.

CHAPTER 1 – YOGA ORIGIN AND SIGNIFICANCE

'Yoga' does not sound like it is a word of English origin, and this implies that the activity did not originate in an English-speaking nation. As a matter of fact, Yoga originated in the regions of ancient India. The word 'yoga' is taken from the Sanskrit root 'yug' which means union. The ultimate goal of yoga is to achieve union between the individual consciousness and the universal divine.

The initial purpose for the practice of Yoga was in no way related to weight loss -weight was not much of a priority for the ancestors. Hindu monks practiced Yoga as a way of attaining a deeper awareness of the self, as well as obtain a degree of inner peace that leads to oneness with a higher entity or the Supreme Being, depending on the person's beliefs.

The Three Main Principles of Yoga

The positions involved in practicing Yoga were built under three main principles:

- *Exercise*

  The postures involve various exercise routines, specifically stretching. This stretching exercise focus mainly on optimizing the strength of the central nervous system especially the lower portion of the spinal column. Ancient Yogis believed that the center of all human consciousness lies at the bottom of the spine that is in the pelvic area.

- *Breathing*

  Most of the techniques used in Yoga postures that focus on breathing are done under the assumption that the breath is the primary life source of all things on earth. The postures often require the Yogi to breathe in deeply and exhale slowly for a couple of minutes or for as long as the Yogi can handle it.

- *Meditation*

  Ancient Yogis believed that meditation is the final step towards achieving that state of total self-awareness and oneness with the Divine. This is the reason why meditation has always been performed at the end of every Yoga session, never before the session or while in the middle of it.

Among these three principles, meditation is probably the most difficult to learn and would take a long time for Yoga practitioners to perfect. This is especially true with today's Yoga practitioners whose minds are cluttered with thoughts of various worries that characterize this century's materialistic culture. However, difficult though it may be to get into a meditative state, it is not an impossible task.

The combination of these three principles effectively ensures that both the body and the mind are involved in the practice of Yoga. And the physical fitness that often results from regular performance of the various Yoga postures often result in a better sense of well-being. This cooperation between the mind and the body is the key towards achieving oneness with the soul and the Higher Being.

The Many Benefits of Yoga

Aside from improved self-awareness, Yoga provides many other benefits, which includes:

- Physical advantages include the development of a leaner and more flexible physique. And because the Yoga postures involve stretching the various parts of the body for long periods, the Yoga practitioner eventually develops stronger muscles.

- The breathing exercises eventually promote a better state of mind. It is actually a well-known fact that breathing deeply in times of crisis or during a state of extreme anger can effectively bring down the person's blood pressure level and bring the heart rate back to normal. This means that the blood being supplied to the brain is within the normal range, thereby promoting calmness and peace of mind.

- Yoga practitioners experience a gradual increase in their intuition. It is a well-known fact that anxiety often reduces a person's capacity for thinking clearly. This means that the individual also tends to lose touch with his inner intuitive self. And, because Yoga promotes a feeling of deep relaxation through the release of stress from the body, the individual starts to renew the connection between his conscious and subconscious self, thereby re-awakening his intuition.

- Yoga also promotes the decrease in pulse rate. This means that Yoga practitioners are less prone to sudden nervous attacks or palpitations.

- Yoga postures also help increase the range of motion for the joints. This also means that Yoga practitioners suffer less from joint pains that are characteristics of rheumatoid arthritis. Aside from this, Yoga also effectively alleviates the painful symptoms of various illnesses.

Yogis also believe that practicing Yoga connects the individual to his own spirituality. Through this connection, Yoga practitioners eventually obtain a better understanding of their place within the circle of life, as well as understand the value of their relationships with fellow humans. These advantages are probably the reasons why many of the biggest names in Hollywood have joined the bandwagon for Yoga as their primary form of physical fitness routine.

CHAPTER 2 - HOW YOGA PROMOTES WEIGHT LOSS

Another well-known fact is that Hollywood celebrities are deeply conscious about their weight. The fact that Yoga promotes the loss of fat in every vital area of the body is probably one more reason why celebrities have become full-pledged Yogis. After all, who wouldn't be interested in obtaining Holistic health by just performing a single exercise method?

However, the more pressing question that probably plagues the minds of people who have not tried Yoga yet is this: How can the stretching exercises involved in the Yoga postures promote weight loss in any part of the body? The answers to this question can be obtained by taking a deeper look at each of the Yoga postures that have been credited to promote weight loss.

Yoga Asanas: Yoga Postures

Listed below are the types of postures and the corresponding organ in the body that each posture takes focuses on:

1. Back-bending postures

This includes the following poses:

* Cobra pose or Bhujangasana

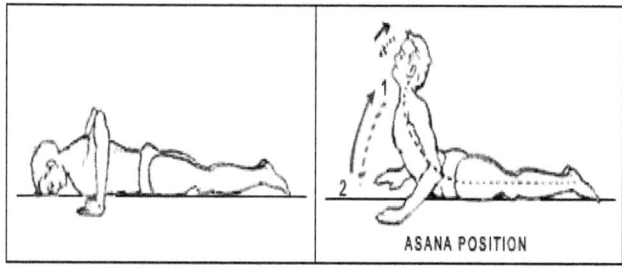

* Bow pose or Dhanurasana

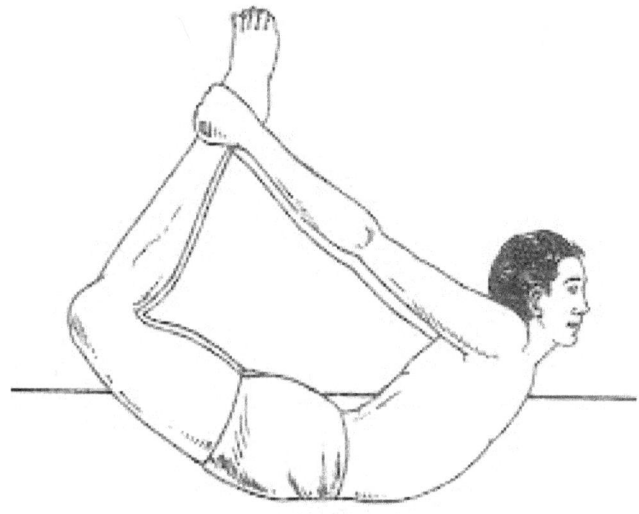

* Spinal Twist or Matsyendrasana

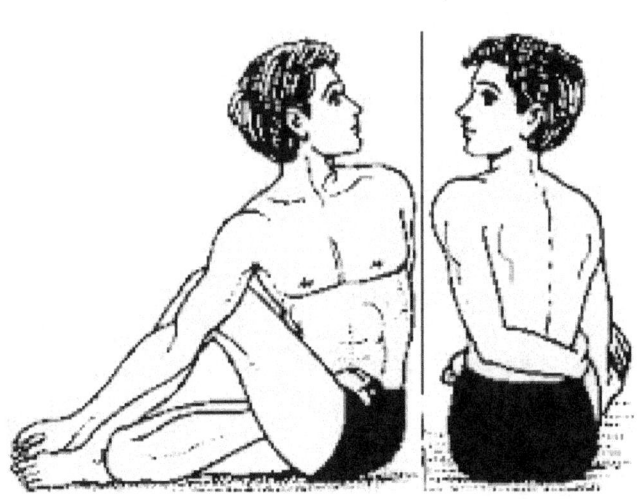

* Wheel pose or Chakrasana

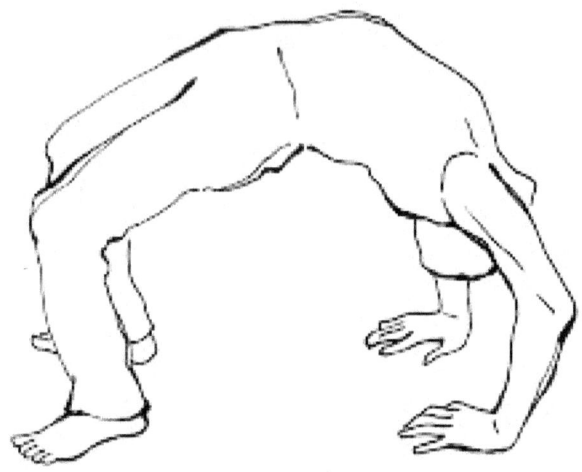

These asanas involve bending the back in one way or another. By doing these poses, the liver is activated and strengthened. This means that the liver becomes healthier, obtaining more energy to cleanse the body of harmful elements, as well as to conduct all of its essential functions with relative ease.

The detoxifying quality of a healthy liver means that fat storage in the abdominal area is at a minimum since the liver effectively burns the excess fat.

2. Seating postures

The Yoga postures that require the practitioner to stretch different parts of the body, normally the limbs and neck, while seated have been proven to be effective in promoting the normal levels of acidity in the body. One of the best-known seating postures is the Paschimottanasana.

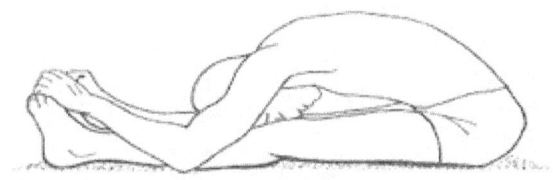

This pose involves sitting on the Yoga mat with both legs extended straight out and the toes of both feet pointing towards the ceiling. The Yogi then extends both hands straight up, bringing the palms of each hand together in the gesture of prayer. Once the arms are fully stretched, the practitioner then elongates the spine in the same manner as the arms.

Both the arms and the upper body should then be brought down into a deep bowing position until the head almost touches the legs. While in this pose, it is important for the practitioner to keep the spine as ramrod straight as possible.

This asana or Yoga posture has almost the same result as doing regular sit-ups at the gym, and that is the creation of rock-hard abs over a period of time. But more than the abs, this pose is essential in stretching the hamstrings and the backbone, making these body parts stronger and more flexible. This pose is also effective in relieving the symptoms of digestive problems and spinal problems such as sciatica. This pose is also effective in the activation of the Yogi's internal body heat because blood is able to flow directly to the brain without any obstructions.

3. The Anjaneyasana (Lunging pose)

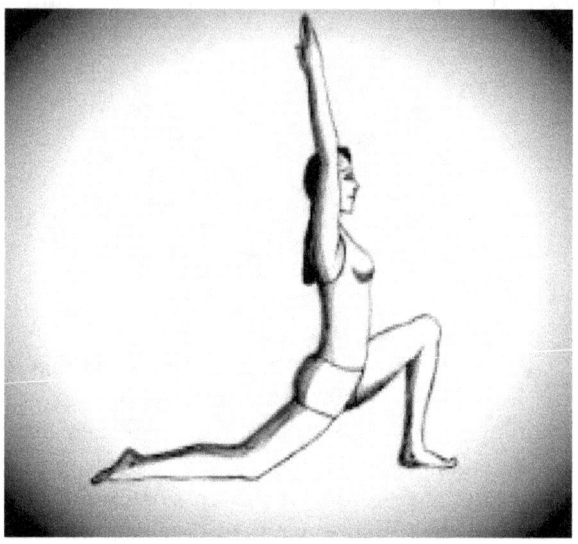

The Anjaneyasana or lunging pose is another pose that promotes the activation of internal body heat because the spinal nerves are stretched and they eventually become taut with tension.

The internal heat generated by this pose eventually works to burn down the deep layers of fat that are more commonly known as subcutaneous fat. Aside from its fat-burning and heat-generating benefits, this asana is also effective in strengthening the quadriceps and the muscles in the butt. The stamina of the lower portion of the body, specifically the thighs, is also improved.

Aside from these three, almost every other Yoga pose promotes weight loss in every part of the human body. Many beginners in the practice of Yoga have been amazed at the amount of sweat produced in their bodies throughout the entire Yoga sessions.

The effort of holding the poses for long periods of time promotes the gradual burning of the subcutaneous fat in the part of the body that is involved in the stretched pose. For instance, during standing poses wherein the legs have to be stretched or the knees bent, the fat in the legs would gradually be melted down.

Likewise, poses that require you to hold hands in stretched positions enables you to strengthen the biceps and other arm muscles while getting rid of excess fat. And because performing the Yoga poses involves stretching all the parts of the body, including the neck, at one time or another, this means that the subcutaneous fat in all of these parts are burned.

Ever noticed how Hindu monks don't seem to have a single ounce of excess fat in any part of their bodies? This is because Yoga is an inherent part of their monkhood. This is a testament to the way that Yoga promotes wellness in the entire human body.

M.E. Dahkid

CHAPTER 3 - UNDERSTANDING STRESS

The definition of the word stress is understood as the state of strain often felt mentally and emotionally that is caused by an external factor or circumstances. Unrelieved stress can cause a buildup over time and eventually lead to further issues with the individual's health and state of mind.

This is why many experts in the medical field, especially psychologists, have recently shifted their focus towards understanding the causes for stress and anxiety, relieving its symptoms, and suggesting ways for avoiding the gradual buildup.

Common Stress Factors

Some of the primary causal factors for stress that experts have identified include:

- *Personal Issues*

Problems that tend to plague the individual's personal life. This includes the death of loved ones, marital or familial issues, and conflict with others with regard to personal beliefs. In the US today, the most common cause of stress for people is the occurrence of an abrupt change in family dynamics, specifically divorce.

Chronic health issues have also been known to cause stress in many individuals. The lack of focus in treating these issues in an individual's personal life have often led people to doing drastic actions, and has been the cause for the increase in the number of people who undergo psychotherapy.

- *Social Issues*

Social issues are considered as secondary factors that affect the individual's level of stress. The most common social stressor is the environment wherein the individual lives. Neighborhoods that provide little security for its dwellers tend to have residents with high stress levels.

Other social situations that could possibly cause stress include the lack of sufficient financial capacity to pay for the individual's needs. In most cases, the lack of funds to pay for the needs of the children in the family has been known to cause a lot of stress for parents.

- *Work Related Issues*

Work problems have also been cited as reasons why people often become stressed and undergo feeling of extreme anxiety. Feelings of inadequacy in performing tasks at work, dissatisfaction with the way things are going at work, and feeling pressured to provide exemplary outputs are some of the problems that career-oriented people often have to deal with at work. Though many people just learn how to deal with these problems and try to endure it for as long as they can, it is not uncommon to hear of workers who have switched to other fields of specialization.

These switchers often find themselves involved in a new industry that has always been in line with their childhood interests and has eventually provided them with more joy in their lives. Although switching to another job that is within one's interests is effective in releasing the pent-up stress, this option is not always possible for every single malcontent employee. This is where the need for stress-reducing activities comes in.

Dealing with Stress

In the same way that feelings of stress slowly builds up over time, the intensity of the stressors also tend to build if it is not addressed early on. Stress often leads people to behavior that may appear stress-inducing on the surface but actually have negative long-term effects for the individual. Some of the most common unhealthy ways that people deal with stress include:

- *Smoking*

Recent surveys have shown that a huge number of nicotine-addicted smokers belong to industries that have the highest levels of stress-inducing factors. This includes people who work at customer service hotlines, research facilities, and the like.

- *Drinking*

Alcoholic drinks in gradually increasing amounts. Many people have turned into alcoholics due to unresolved feelings of stress.

- *Gambling*

In most instances, the individual may start out by betting a few pennies here and there. This could lead to big-time gambling activities that can drown a person in piles of debt, which would defeat the purpose for gambling since debt tends to increase stress.

- *Withdrawal from social situations.*

Social withdrawal is avoiding people and activities you would usually enjoy; for some people, this can progress to a point of social isolation, where you may even want to avoid contact with family and close friends and just be by yourself most of the time. You may want to be alone because you feel it's tiring or upsetting to be with other people.

- *A growing interest or disinterest in food.*

This means that the individual may gradually become obese or underweight.

These unhealthy options for dealing with stress have become so prevalent in recent years that many of the world's leading health organizations have become alarmed. In this atmosphere of unhealthy lifestyles, the proponents have luckily been able to gain success in educating the populace about Yoga and how it can serve as the best method for stress reduction.

One of Yoga's most notable contributions to stress-reduction is the fact that the Yoga postures also involve the regulation of breathing while the practitioner stays in each asana for as long as he could endure to do so. There are also several postures that require nothing more than sitting still while breathing deeply in and out.

The final routine in Yoga exercises, which is meditation, has also been dubbed as the best form of mind relaxation ever invented. And having a relaxed mind is tantamount to having a stress-free mind.

M.E. Dahkid

CHAPTER 4- YOGA POSES FOR STRESS-REDUCTION

Although the entire Yoga session results in an overall feeling of relaxation and stress is released all throughout, there are a few postures that have been credited to reduce a higher amount of stress as compared to the other postures. There are at least 10 of these postures, and the list includes the following:

1. *The salutation posture*

The salutation posture (also known as Pramasan or Anjali Mudra.) Aside from being a Yoga asana or posture, this stance is also universally known as a posture that denotes respect.

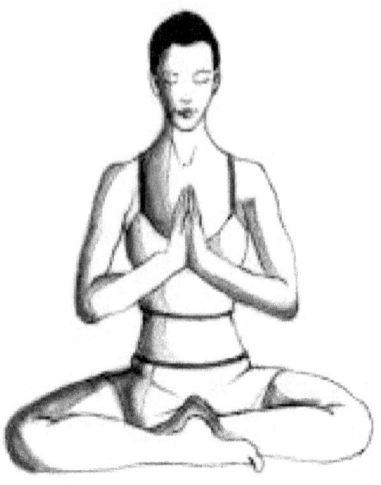

Hindus often use this pose in greeting each other, and it is also an inherent form of the greeting gestures in other cultures. This pose can be done by bringing the palm of each hand to the chest area and then pressing both together with the fingers fully extended upward.

This pose is not only used for greeting, it is also used in saying goodbye. When used as a Yoga asana, the practitioner has to be comfortably seated with the legs crossed.

This asana is effective in releasing stress because it brings the Yogi into a state of meditative self-awareness. Yogis also believe that this pose effectively balances the left and right dimensions of personality, harmonizing these two in the middle where the heart chakra is located.

2. *The so-called 'Easy' pose*

Known in the ancient Yoga tradition as Sukhasana, this pose is relaxing not only for adult Yoga practitioners but also to children since the pose is often done by kids unconsciously during playtime.

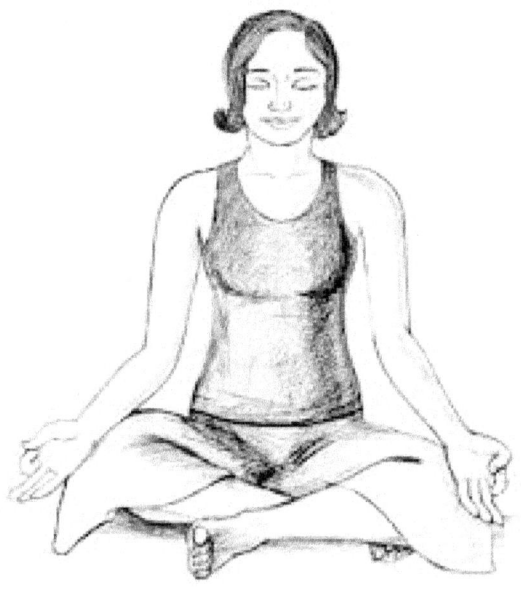

This pose is highly stress-reducing because of the way that the nerves are gradually soothed through constant repetition of Sukhasana.

Constantly doing the Easy pose also results in the loosening up of the hip and thigh muscles, two areas of the body that often feel the most strain due to sitting in an office chair for 8 or more hours a day. Once the muscles are loosened up, individuals often feel more relaxed and are less prone to pain in that area.

Sukhasana falls under the category of Yoga postures known as 'sitting' poses. In order to perform this asana, the practitioner has to first sit on the Yoga mat in a relaxed position. He then has to stretch both legs straight out. He should then bring both feet inwards until the legs are crossed in a triangle.

A marked difference between this pose and other sitting postures is that in Sukhasana, there is a slight gap between the pelvic bones and feet whereas other sitting postures require the feet to be tucked in underneat the pelvic area.

Beginners may find this pose difficult to perform on their first few tries, and this is something that could cause a little bit more stress. However, with constant repetition could cause the muscles to gradually relax and make the pose easier to perform. This is when the stress-reducing effect of Sukhasana can be felt.

3. *Uttana Shishosana*

Also known as the Extended Dog or Stretching Dog pose.

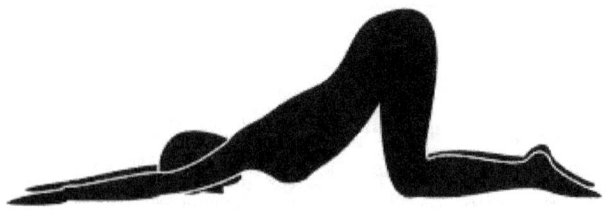

This pose is highly effective in reducing tension because of the way that it calms the practitioner's mind and releases tension in the neck, the back and the head. This pose has also been known to cure cases of chronic insomnia.

The Uttana Shishosana pose is among the Yoga poses that are highly recommended for employees who sit in the office for very long hours. This is because sitting can cause too much tension in the back and the hips. This tension is often manifested as muscle pain in the lower back and in the butt muscles.

This pose can be performed by first going down on all fours, imitating the stance of a dog. It is important to make sure that the shoulders are aligned with the wrists, and the hips are aligned with the knees. With the palm of both hands lying flat on the floor, the Yogi would then have to move his hands a few inches to the front. The butt should then be moved back towards the heels while keeping both hands right where they are.

The elbows should not touch the floor at any time during this pose. Keeping the neck relaxed, the forehead has to be dropped down until it touches the mat. Make sure that the back is slightly curved and then stretch the arms a little bit further and lowering the butt down further towards the heels. Breathe in and out deeply while maintaining the pose for as long as possible.

4. *The Cow pose or Bitilasana*

The first step for this pose is quite similar with the Uttana Shishoasna wherein the practitioner is in a dog-like position with the shoulders, wrists, hips, and knees properly aligned. The next step involves bringing the head into a central position with the eyes looking downwards.

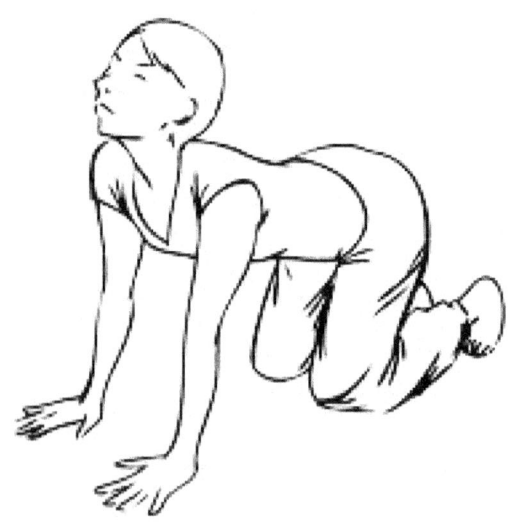

The practitioner should then lift the chest and pelvic bones upward while dipping the stomach down. This step has to be done during inhalation of breath. Next step is to lift the head until the eyes are looking directly forward. Release the position upon exhalation. The suggested number of repetitions for this step is around 10 to 20 times per session.

The Bitilasana is considered a stress-reducing pose because it has the same calming effect as the other asanas on this list. Aside from this, Bitilasana is also known to neutralize the emotions, making it more balanced through the proper flow of blood to the heart and up the spine to the brain.

This asana is also known to stimulate the proper functioning of the various organs inside the stomach, including the adrenal glands and the kidneys. This improvement in the health of the abdominal area is sure to bring more peace of mind to the practitioner, thereby promoting peace of mind and the reduction of stress.

5. The Forward Bend while seated pose or Pascimottanasana.

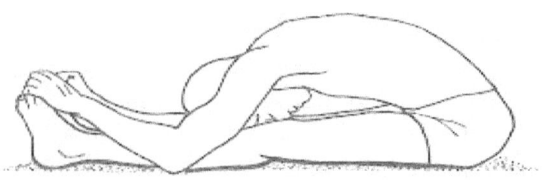

(Mentioned previously in the weight-loss poses) This pose may look like it is easy to perform, but beginners might encounter difficulties especially if they have pot bellies. Out of all the stress-reducing Yoga postures, this one is probably the only one that has a lot of benefits for numerous organs in the body. These benefits include:

- Stretching the hamstrings
- Stretching the spine, as well as the lower back
- Promotes a marked improvement in digestion
- Relieves the painful symptoms of dysmenorrhea or PMS (pre-menstual syndrome)
- Stimulates the proper functioning of the internal organs in the abdomen. This includes the uterus and the ovaries.

This pose can be performed by first sitting on the floor in a relaxed position while keeping the spine straight. As the English name of this asana indicates, the rest of the steps required for this pose involve bending the torso forward until the forehead touches the knees.

Apparently, based on the asanas or postures listed above, the best Yoga postures that promote relaxation involve sitting and stretching the spine. This is enough proof of the fact that tension in the spine, whether it is in the lower or upper back, is the primary reason why stress sets in.

Experts also suggest that a tensed backbone and pelvic area, including tension in the abdominal area, hinders the proper flow of blood to the brain. This means that the brain suffers from lack of oxygen, thereby causing the aches and pains associated with stress such as migraine.

M.E. Dahkid

CHAPTER 5 – YOGA'S ROLE IN FINDING INNER PEACE

Many people were surprised when the first few Hollywood celebrities came out and announced that Yoga was their primary fitness routine. The articles were often met with skepticism since Yoga was better known as a Hindu practice of meditation. However, as more and more celebrities, including fitness experts and health gurus, joined the bandwagon, more information about the extensive benefits of Yoga started to be notice by everyday people.

Nowadays, it is common for a fitness gym to offer Yoga classes as part of their fitness routines. Yoga has even evolved into sessions that have been customized for the specific needs of the practitioners such as Yoga sessions that are specifically tailored for pregnant women. Many of the testimonies from Yoga practitioners include statements such as:

- A marked improvement in the way that people

handled negative and stressful situations in their lives.

- A shift in focus from the negative aspects of life to the positive.

- A marked improvement in sleeping patterns. Many insomniacs have reported that they were able to fall asleep at night without the ingesting any sleeping medication as soon as they started practicing Yoga.

- The typical aches and pains that are associated with living stressful lives have all disappeared.

Is Yoga Really The Answer?

Many practitioners have also reported that their personal relationships benefited the most out of their Yoga sessions. This is because their positive outlooks are manifested in the way they deal with conflicts, as well as in the way they cope with stressful situations. But what makes Yoga special? More importantly, how does an exercise routine that involves a lot of stretching, bending back and forth, and deep breathing help a practitioner find inner peace?

The answer to these questions is simple: the different Yoga postures promote the proper functioning of the organs in the body. What does a healthily functioning organ mean? It means that the individual is able to get all the nutrients that he needs for performing various tasks because these nutrients have been distributed evenly throughout the body by the healthy organs. It also means that hormones are properly regulated, providing very little cause for the development of hormone-related illnesses.

Yoga postures also strengthen the muscles over time, and this means that practitioners are able to perform their daily tasks with more ease.

On the same note, Yoga also serves as a catalyst for finding inner peace because all of its postures promote the rapid burning of excess fat in the parts of the body involved in each posture.

For instance, the sitting postures such as the Paschimottanasana are effective in burning excess fat in the abdominal and pelvic area; the standing postures effectively burn off the excess fat in the arms and legs, and so on.

Because of this fat-burning mechanism, Yoga practitioners often find themselves leaner and more physically fit within just a few months of practicing Yoga. And it is no secret that physical fitness is almost equivalent to mental and emotional fitness since physically fit people have a very small chance of getting bullied.

Physical fitness also means that the individual is less prone to illnesses that are common among obese individuals such as diabetes and high blood pressure. In this way, Yoga promotes the achievement of inner peace for the individual.

Aside from all these, another way that Yoga can promote inner peace is because it involves meditation. Ancient Yogis believed that 'prana' flows more freely throughout the body when the individual is in a state of deep relaxation, a state that is now referred to as meditation. For the sake of clarity, prana is defined as the 'life-force', the culmination of all the energy flowing within the cosmic universe. It is believed that the energy starts from the sun and flows through all living things, connecting them. Prana is said to be the force that is responsible for the maintenance of heat and life in the body of a human being. It is a bit difficult to find a scientific equivalent for prana in the modern world.

Moving on, ancient Yogis believed that meditation promotes the proper flow of prana in the body, thereby shielding the individual from harmful elements that could cause illness and diseases. A recent study has proven this belief to be correct, and this means that Yoga is now supported by solid scientific evidence. In that study, it was found that Yoga practitioners had an active gene that is responsible for fending diseases off. This gene was not found in the lab samples for individuals who did not practice any form of stress-reducing exercise.

CHAPTER 6 – HOW MEDITATION IS BENEFICIAL FOR YOGA PRACTITIONERS

Yoga practitioners who are always on the go often find it difficult to master the art of meditation on their first tries. This is because meditation requires the supreme act of sitting very still and trying not to dash back and forth because of forgotten chores or answering the phone.

The practitioner has to commit himself to doing absolutely nothing, as opposed to the way that he is expected to do everything at work or at home. In order for meditation to be successful, it requires the person to free himself from consciously steering his thoughts by not thinking of all the tasks that need to be accomplished and simply allowing the thoughts to flow freely.

The meditative state can be reached faster by linking the mind to the process of breathing. This can be done by trying to visualize the breath that comes in during each inhalation and try to see the air that is going out upon exhalation. It might also help if the individual concentrates on the sounds all around him instead of concentrating on his thoughts.

The benefit of opening the ears to the surroundings is

twofold: it frees the mind for meditation, and it increases the individual's attentiveness to everything around him.

Advantages of Meditation

The advantages of meditation are extensive and these have been categorized into 3 main groups:

1. De-stressing benefits –

This involves two factors: the prevention of stress from invading the mind, and the release of all the pent-up stress from the mind and the body. These two things happen at the same time while the individual is meditating. This means that after meditation, Yoga practitioners becomes more relaxed and feel more joyful and positive. These positive feelings then lead to the achievement of inner peace.

2. Physical benefits –

The list is long and it includes the lowering of blood pressure for hypertensive individuals, a marked reduction of anxiety attacks, a marked improvement in the functioning of the immune system. Yoga practitioners also experience a marked increase in their positive moods because of the effect of meditation in increasing the levels of serotonin released in the brain.

3. Mental benefits –

The primary benefit that meditation brings to the mental health of Yoga practitioners is the way that it brings the brainwaves up to the Alpha state. Under normal circumstances, Alpha waves are only present when the individual is in a relaxed state such as when the eyes are closed in wakeful relaxation. Alpha waves are significant because they promote the rapid healing of tissues throughout the body.

These brainwaves are also credited for the creativeness of artists and the focused attention of marksmen on their targets. By accessing these waves through meditation, Yoga practitioners end up with feelings of contentment wherein they are less prone to feelings of powerfully negative emotions. This is probably the reason why Hindu monks are always so calm and retrospective.

An Ancient Belief

Ancient Yogis believed that the physical exercises, the stretching and back bending, are all required actions that prepare the individual for the final state of Yoga. That the flow of prana in the backbone and throughout the body is a necessary step in preparing the individual for the act of freeing his mind from all clutter. There is a reason why meditation always comes at the end of each Yoga session.

This is because through meditation, the consciousness of Yoga practitioners evolves until they eventually become ready for the higher form of consciousness, also known as the cosmic consciousness.

Cosmic consciousness, or the Fifth state of Consciousness, is believed to be the individual's awareness that everything in the universe is one and the understanding that everything is interconnected. Cosmic consciousness is believed to be the foundation for mysticism and the oneness of the universe.

Because the aspects of cosmic consciousness are often contradictory to the teachings of leading religions about the presence of one God who rules over everything, it is often unacceptable for some people, even if they are hardcore Yoga practitioners. This is probably the reason why there are so few people alive today who have managed to attain this fifth state in the level of their consciousness despite the proliferation of Yoga and other meditation techniques.

A FINAL WORD

Practicing yoga promotes peace. When you slow down and tune in to yourself, you feel more confident, less stressed, stronger, and free from negativity. It truly is being good to yourself; it is your gift to yourself. Take that feeling and share it with others. It is easier to be nice to people when you feel good, physically and mentally.

I want to take this time out to thank you for purchasing this book! The next step is to take action on the advice you've just read about.

Please Leave a Review

Finally, if you enjoyed this book, please take the time to share your thoughts and post a review on Amazon. It'd be greatly appreciated!

That review and feedback will help me improve the content in my books – and make each and every one more relevant and helpful to you.

Thank you again and good luck!

M.E. Dahkid